Chocolate Smoothies
by Ibsen Bjorn G.

Get All The Books In The Series:

Table of Contents

8. The Cherry Chocolate Smoothie.

9. The Chocolate Raspberry love affair.

10. The Bahama Coconut Chocolate Sunset.

11. The Chocolate Strawberry Smoothie.

12. The Chocolate Coffee Smoothie.

13. The Frauline (German Chocolate Smoothie).

14. The French Silk Pie Smoothie.

15. The Chocolate Caramel Smoothie.

INTRODUCTION-

Welcome to the Chocolate Smoothies recipe book. This ebook contains recipes for various smoothies that are not only chocolaty, but also considerably healthy. Each one has some nutritional value, and will be fun to try (and retry).

We live in a world that's growing more and more health conscious. But sometimes it seems like going the healthy route means giving up the tastes we love. This book shows… that's not necessarily true.

Some recipes in this book include flax seeds, nuts and other such ingredients that must be well blended, so it is recommended that a high-power blender be used, such as a vitamix, blendtec, nutribullet or other comparable blender.

Step out of the ordinary with these ideas and see how a dab of creativity can add a whole lot of flavor to your world. Whether it's for yourself or for a party, a date night or a dessert, there aren't many situations that a chocolate smoothie can't make better.

Let's move forward now to the real reason we're here. The smoothies.

1. The Peanut Butter/Chocolate Slow Dance.

Ingredients:

½ cup 2% milk
2 tablespoons chocolate syrup
2 tablespoons peanut butter of your choice
1 Avocado
½ cup ice
1 (8-ounce) package of vanilla yogurt

Preparation:

1. Place all ingredients into a high powered blender and blend until smooth.
2. Pour into your favorite smoothie drinking container.
3. Enjoy!

2. The Chocolate Almond Escape.

Ingredients:

1 cup of kefir
A pinch of sea salt
1 tablespoon cacao nibs
1 avocado (peeled and de-seeded)
2 tablespoons of almond butter
½ teaspoon vanilla extract
Approximately 1 tablespoon of honey (sweetener)
4 ice cubes
1/4 teaspoon cinnamon
1/2 cup almond milk
1 cup of spinach
1 tablespoon of flax seeds

1 tablespoon of colostrum (optional)
1 tablespoon spirulina

Preparation:

1. Place all ingredients into a high powered blender and blend until smooth.
2. Pour into your favorite smoothie drinking container.
3. Enjoy!

3. The Dark Dream.

Ingredients:

1 cup chocolate frozen yogurt
2 tablespoons unsweetened cocoa
1/2 cup sweetened coconut milk
Dark chocolate shavings for garnish

Preparation:

1. Place all ingredients into a high powered blender and blend until smooth.
2. Pour into your favorite smoothie drinking container.
3. Garnish with chocolate shavings.

4. Enjoy!

4. The Chocolate Fudge Smoothie.

Ingredients:

1 cup of 2% milk
2 tsp cocoa powder
2 tbsp chocolate protein powder
1 Large Avocado
A pinch of salt
1/4 tsp pure vanilla extract
½ cup chocolate almond milk
2 tbsp almond butter

Preparation:

1. Place all ingredients into a high powered blender and blend until smooth.
2. Pour into your favorite smoothie drinking container.
3. Enjoy!

5. The Chocolate Mint Smoothie.

Ingredients:

1 cup nonfat Greek yogurt
1/4 cup fresh mint
1 cup almond milk
2 cups ice
¼ cup dark chocolate chips
1 cup of fresh, green spinach
1 tablespoon honey

Preparation:

1. Place all ingredients into a high powered blender and blend until smooth.

2. Pour into your favorite smoothie drinking container.
3. Enjoy!

6. The Chocolate Peppermint Smoothie.

Ingredients:

1½ cups sweetened coconut milk
1 avocado
2 tablespoons unsweetened cocoa powder
1 tablespoon honey
2 teaspoons peppermint extract
1 cup fresh, green spinach
1 tablespoon flax seeds
8 ice cubes
2 tablespoons fresh mint

Preparation:

1. Place all ingredients into a high powered blender and blend until smooth.
2. Pour into your favorite smoothie drinking container.
3. Top with whipped cream.
4. Garnish with mint.
5. Serve and enjoy!

7. The Chocolate Banana Smoothie

Ingredients:

8 ice cubes
1 cup unsweetened coconut milk
1 banana
½ cup chocolate chips
1 teaspoon vanilla extract
1 tablespoon honey

Preparation:

1. Place all ingredients into a high powered blender and blend until smooth.

2. Pour into your favorite smoothie consuming vessel.
3. Serve and enjoy!

8. The Cherry Chocolate Smoothie.

Ingredients:

1 avocado
½ frozen banana
1 cup of frozen cherries
1 tbsp of cocoa powder
1 scoop of chocolate protein powder
6 oz of unsweetened almond milk
¼ tsp of almond extract
1 handful of fresh, green spinach

Preparation:

1. Place all ingredients into a high powered blender and blend until smooth.
2. Pour into your favorite smoothie consuming vessel.
3. Garnish with extra frozen cherries.
4. Serve and enjoy!

9. The Chocolate Raspberry love affair.

Ingredients:

1 cup of Yogurt (plain or vanilla)
3/4 to 1 cup vanilla coconut milk
1 cup frozen raspberries
1 avocado
1 Tablespoon honey
2 tablespoons unsweetened cocoa powder
1 square of 60% cacao dark chocolate from a 4 oz. bar, for garnish

Preparation:

1. Place all ingredients (except for garnish) into a high powered blender and blend until smooth.
2. Pour into your favorite smoothie consuming vessel.
3. Add 3 frozen raspberries as a garnish on top.
4. Chop dark chocolate into shreds and garnish on top.
5. Serve and enjoy!

10. The Bahama Coconut Chocolate Sunset.

Ingredients:

½ cup canned coconut milk
1 cup unsweetened coconut milk
¼ cup unsweetened cocoa powder
½ cup melted coconut oil
1 small handful spinach
½ cup flax seeds
¼ cup agave nectar

Preparation:

1. Place all ingredients into a high powered blender and blend until smooth.

2. Pour into your favorite smoothie consuming vessel.
3. Serve and enjoy!

11. The Chocolate Strawberry Smoothie.

Ingredients:

2 bananas, frozen and chunked
1/2 cup frozen strawberries
2 tablespoons chocolate syrup
1 cup plain yogurt

Preparation:

1. Place all ingredients into a high powered blender and blend until smooth.
2. Pour into your favorite smoothie consuming vessel.
3. Serve and enjoy!

12. The Chocolate Coffee Smoothie.

Ingredients:

3 cups brewed coffee
1 avocado
1 banana
1/2 cup hemp protein powder
1/2 cup almonds
2 tsps vanilla extract
1 tsp cinnamon

Preparation:

1. Place all ingredients into a high powered blender and blend until smooth.

2. Pour into your favorite smoothie consuming vessel.
3. Serve and enjoy!

13. The Frauline (German Chocolate Smoothie).

Ingredients:

3 Tbs pecans
1 Tbs flaxseed
2 Tbs carob chips
2 Tbs shredded coconut
¼ tsp cardomom
¼ tsp nutmeg
½ tsp vanilla extract
½ cup frozen pineapple
½ cup apple
½ banana (frozen)
1 cup of coconut milk
3 ice cubes

Preparation:

1. Place all ingredients into a high powered blender and blend until smooth.
2. Pour into your favorite smoothie consuming vessel.
3. Sprinkle some Granola on top as a garnish.
4. Serve and enjoy!

14. The French Silk Pie Smoothie.

Ingredients:

½ cup chocolate protein powder
1 tablespoon rolled oats
1 cup chocolate almond milk
4 ice cubes
1 tablespoon unsweetened baking cocoa
1 teaspoon vanilla
1 tablespoon frozen (thawed) fat-free whipped topping
1 whole graham cracker rectangle
1 teaspoon grated bittersweet chocolate

Preparation:

1. Place all ingredients into a high powered blender and blend until smooth.
2. Pour into your favorite smoothie consuming vessel.
3. Serve and enjoy!

15. The Chocolate Caramel Smoothie.

Ingredients:

1 cup coconut water
1 frozen banana
2 Tbsp. raw cacao powder
12 macadamia nuts (shelled)
1 date (pitted)
2 tsp. coconut sugar
Pinch sea salt
5 ice cubes

Preparation:

1. Place all ingredients into a high powered blender and blend until smooth.
2. Pour into your favorite smoothie consuming vessel.
3. Serve and enjoy!

Get All The Books In The Series:

The Paleo Pocket Breakfast Partner
The Paleo Pocket Dinner Partner